Table of Contents

The Benefits of Walking for Relieving Back Pain

1. Introduction to Back Pain and Walking

1.1. Understanding Back Pain

1.2. Benefits of Walking for Back Pain Relief

The Effects of Walking on Back Pain: A Comprehensive Review

1. Introduction

Walking is popular, well-tolerated, accessible, and typically has fewer barriers to the initiation of exercise than any other form of exertion, both standard and more sophisticated. Here, we conduct a comprehensive review of experimental studies that have enrolled adults with back pain and have been asked to walk as part of a research study intervention. We searched a range of literature databases and included relevant papers in our overview. This is the first review of its kind, and we direct our focus exclusively to walking, as distinct from other forms of exercise. The rest of our essay is organized meticulously to study this topic in depth.

The experience of back pain affects people around the world and has immense financial implications, both for individuals managing care costs and for society at large. Alleviating the symptoms of back pain would improve the health, quality of life, and overall productivity of everyone. Regular exercise is one of the non-invasive interventions that have strong scientific evidence in its favor, and it is recommended as part of the standard care pathway by a number of international guidelines.

1.1. Background and Significance

This review will consider the psychological state, as well as walking gait and features, and pain and physical function outcomes, of people with back pain. Walking is a common, low-impact mode of aerobic exercise that has been suggested to have beneficial effects on back pain at various time frames and has been recommended for people with back pain in clinical practice guidelines. Clarification regarding the effectiveness of walking (versus no intervention or alternative treatments), as well as the potential for walking parameters, strategies, gait patterns, or features to aid in predicting therapeutic response or aid in the development of precision medicine for people with walking is unclear. Symposium - University of Minnesota, St. Paul, MN, USA.

Background and significance: Spinal pain is one of the most common and costly health conditions. Recurrence of spinal pain is also common. Physical inactivity and low cardiorespiratory capacity are associated with the onset of back pain and poor recovery. Many interventions are available for back pain, including treatments for non-specific back pain, such as manual therapy or exercise. Exercise, which includes aerobic exercise, to reduce back pain and improve cardiorespiratory fitness has been clinically recommended. Walking is a common form of aerobic activity, and it has been proposed that walking has many benefits, such as improving pain. However, the nature and magnitude of the effects of walking on back pain have not yet been comprehensively reviewed.

2. Anatomy and Mechanisms of Back Pain

2.1. Anatomy of the Spine

2.2. Common Causes of Back Pain

2.3. Mechanisms of Pain Perception

3. Benefits of Walking on Back Health

Walking supports the flow of nutrient-rich fluids. Vital for the health and correct function of the back is the supply of nutrients—chiefly, via blood—to the tissues of the back. It is reported that walking can help to improve the flow of blood around the body. Furthermore, hydration and intervertebral disc mechanical loading help further stimulate the flow of nutrients to the back during weight-bearing activities, such as walking. The qualitative and quantitative function of healthy spinal intervertebral discs is also reliant on the flow of nutrients and hydration to the disc via the endplates. Compressive movements like walking can positively stimulate the flow of these nutrients into the disc and decrease intervertebral disc thickness (IVD) swelling. Thus, regular movement can promote the movement of essential nutrients and hydration around the spinal column, creating an environment suitable for the body to repair and prevent painful back conditions.

Walking combats sedentary lifestyles. Walking has long been proposed as a means of reversing some of the physically deleterious effects of modern, mostly sedentary, lifestyles and professions. When it comes to the back, our bodies benefit greatly from maintaining appropriate, naturally adapted physical activity and rest patterns. Walking offers a chance for regular postural change, leading to less multi-directional and prolonged static stress on the muscles, ligaments, and joints of the back. In particular, with increased core activation, walking is effective at potentially preventing muscular strength and endurance deficits in the trunk musculature, as reported by both investigations using electromyographic activity of the muscles of the spine and comparable research using trunk muscle cross-sectional areas. Furthermore, walking aids the stretching of the paraspinal musculature with appropriate, safe, repetitive loading. As reported by Usain Bolt, walking can additionally provide a "full-body exercise, depending on the walking style."

3.1. Improvement in Posture

In scoliosis, the importance of gait was highlighted by Schroth, who prioritized an individualized gait rehabilitation programme designed to improve the postural stability of the lumbar spine. Schroth described pointed training towards 'positive shift' walking, supplemented with relaxation techniques and physiotherapy sessions, in line with Vojta, though from a slightly less central muscular concern basis. It is now known that in left lumbar scoliosis, the quadratus lumborum of the left is weaker; walking to the left therefore helps correct the posture somewhat, and other left muscles are then focused on in exercise. Functional gait is taught in the domains of neurology by health-related professionals, even in elderly patients, to improve the dynamic component of posture. Upright posture assisted by walking has become a staple teaching activity in senior care services throughout the world, while introductory aspects of gait rehabilitation have been incorporated into physiotherapy and rehabilitation medicine undergraduate courses in the East.

3.1. Improvement in posture. Many elements of a walking programme have the ability to affect a shift from acute to chronic pain. Notably, acquiring the correct posture when walking, which would usually be considered easier due to the lower energetic requirements and the fact it is a low-intensity cardiovascular exercise (at the correct pace), does not correspond to how easy it is for someone in pain to accomplish (such an individual is very likely holding an individualistic posture to ease pain). Larger strides are recommended in ideal posture and walking that is clearly focused on heels (commonly seen in shorter strides—especially if the individual also ambulates with straight legs) can lead to vertebral movement that significantly increases the amount of anterior-posterior tilting of the pelvis at the initiation of each propulsive stride. However, an upright position while walking tends to activate the multifidi more than a slouched position.

3.2. Strengthening of Core Muscles

Many rehabilitation programs for back pain are designed to increase the strength, endurance, and control of local stabilizing and large prime mover muscles believed to play a role in the development and persistence of back pain (e.g., multifidi, transversus abdominis, and lumbar erector spinae). Walking is not traditionally considered a rehabilitation intervention for this purpose, and many who have reported changes in muscle size, composition, and mechanics that reduced pain and/or prevented back injury due to walking have done so in the context of illness, disease, or injury in muscle populations that differ from those associated with back pain. The synergistic muscles impacted by walking may be even less commonly mentioned in lumbar rehabilitation interventions. For example, Scannell and McGill found that the effects of back pain on muscle activity were curvilinear (u-shaped), but that muscles deeper to the back pain muscles and with passing through the zone of 'comfort' may become active to compensate for the large muscles closer to the spine that had been inhibited by the pain.

3.2. Strengthening of core muscles. The seven studies that discussed walking as a means to increase the strength and/or endurance of core muscles discussed improvements in abdominal or lumbar muscle size, thickness, and fatty infiltration, as well as improvements in musculature cross-sectional area and volume. Additionally, four studies (31%) discussed improvements in dynamic, synergistic muscles such as the psoas and paraspinals, as well as the diaphragm among subsamples. Although the reviewed effects may point to improvements from walking and some benefits may be gained from increased muscle size for back pain, the clinical relevance of muscle size, composition, and endurance is not immediately clear. However, increases in dynamic muscles may decrease the potential for compensatory pain from muscles such as the quadratus lumborum and may further speak to an antalgic gait minimization strategy.

3.3. Increased Blood Flow and Nutrient Delivery

Several researchers have suggested that cardiovascular health could be a predictive factor for persons with LBP to be active and involved in sports at a younger age. Physical activity has a general effect on the cardiovascular system, regardless of what the activity looks like, and it is thus conceivable that the systemic muscles of the lumbar spine are involved in performing the motor programme. Considering the direction of the walking model based on kinematic studies, the load is biased more towards the retractor muscle. That is, the back muscles actively controlling the pelvis suspension are required to be most involved and would seem to benefit from an increased blood flow over time. However, it is still unclear how mechanical factors play a role in metabolism. With an increased flow, healing factors of LBP could actively be transported or promoted. For that matter, there seems to be a gap in the literature about the effects of walking on the back, and future studies are needed.

In contrast to cycling and swimming, walking is associated with increased muscle activity in the lower back, even though the absolute muscular demand may still be low. The increased muscular demand during walking is associated with the biomechanical need to steady and elongate the back to enable free motion in the limbs. In addition to increased muscle activity, walking has been shown to cause substantial compression and decompression of the lumbar vertebrae. These relatively large dynamic changes in pressure may account for the high nociceptive activity during walking found in studies of patients with chronic low back pain (LBP-related pain).

4. Scientific Studies and Evidence

In recent studies, the results are conclusive that walking can result in some improvement in back pain. An intimate hiker submitted the results in the latest systematic review paper. The majority of studies have reported that walking can result in psychological or psychosocial benefits, including reduced disability, depression, anxiety, and fear. The reasoning behind this is that walking is an easy, accessible, and inexpensive way to exercise, and walk and talk therapy is considered effective in reducing stress, anxiety, and aiding in weight loss as well.

Moreover, when a meta-analysis or systematic review provides strong evidence, it is considered a well-powered study. The effectiveness of any intervention that is tested would be applicable to a wide population and not specific to a particular group of people. A test or investigation that is carried out and observed would qualify as strong evidence, and such studies help in creating guidelines or standards for treatment. It is also reasonable to assume that any recommendations made would be applicable to a large group of patients.

Firstly, the scientific evidence that deals with walking and its effect on back pain patients is important. A critical piece of evidence would be a systematic review, which analyzes the data that has been considered up to date. The most trustworthy evidence is considered when it has been compared and validated against various meta-analyses, randomized control trials, and comparative studies. The next level of studies is considered as individual studies that are conducted over a longer period of time. These studies help in understanding the effectiveness of a particular treatment for a specific outcome.

4.1. Systematic Reviews and Meta-Analyses

In general, reviews were funded through governmental and research-based organizations, including the National Health and Medical Research Council (NHMRC, Australia), the Spanish Ministry of Economy and Competitiveness, the Swedish Research Council, the VA Health Services Research and Development (HSRD, USA), and The Netherlands Organisation for Health Research and Development. Conflicting results were reported, with the effect of walking interventions in counts of reviews as for, against, or uncertain. Many of these containing discussion regarding the determination of efficacy for a lack of treatment-related side effects or increased adherence due to the involvement of minimal risk in walking.

Under the guidance of the Preferred Reporting Items for Systematic Reviews and Meta-Analyses (PRISMA) statement, a total of 13 systematic reviews/meta-analyses were identified in relation to walking as a treatment for back pain published in the search period. The search strategy is outlined in Additional file 3, with the corresponding PRISMA flow chart provided in Additional file 4. Among the included systematic reviews/meta-analyses, the etiology of back pain and conditions examined within the reviews included non-specific back pain, scoliosis, ankylosing spondylitis, and lumbar fusion surgery. Reviews further included both acute and chronic cases, with some focusing on post-partum or post-partum populations. One study featured a meta-analysis, pooling results for treatment effects on back pain intensity and disability between studies to create a mean difference in scores for each outcome. Due to this pooling, lower back pain was expected to be evaluated as a continuous variable in this review. Narrative analysis was conducted for all other included reviews, with different outcomes reported for back pain according to study, including visual analog scale (VAS) and numerical rating scale (NRS) for low back pain intensity, physical function, disability, quality of life (QoL), depression, and reduction in fear of re-injury.

4.2. Randomized Controlled Trials

Beales et al. examined the effects of a nonproficiency-based walking program in individuals with lower limb amputation with LBP and aortoiliac disease. Participants randomly assigned to the walking group participated in a 10-week regular practice self-paced walking program, while the passive group of participants refrained from further walking training during the intervention period. A lower level of self-reported leg pain during walking was seen for the passive group directly postoperatively ($p < 0.001$), after 6 months ($p = 0.02$), and at 12 months ($p = 0.002$). At one year, a smaller improvement in back pain self-efficacy was reported in the passive group ($p = 0.047$). No treatment by time interaction effect was found for self-reported CBLP at any time point of the study, but a diminished perception of disability based on the ODI was observed at the 6-month ($p = 0.006$) and 12-months ($p < 0.001$) follow-up.

Randall et al. performed a RCT evaluating the effects of a supervised walking program in patients with CBLP. The walking program consisted of a one-hour session of treadmill and over-ground walking at moderate intensity, three times per week, for 12 weeks. The control group continued their usual care and were given a recommendation to walk for health. In comparison to the control group, no between-group differences were observed in self-reported pain at 11 ($p = 0.12$) or 26 ($p = 0.06$) weeks. The walking group presented greater disability at 11 ($p = 0.048$) and 26 weeks ($p = 0.04$) than the wait-list group, while no between-group difference was seen using the Oswestry Disability Index (ODI).

4.3. Longitudinal Studies

The findings of longitudinal studies that examined the impact of walking on back pain reveal a fascinating model for the relationships between walking and back pain. The most consistent finding that we found from these past studies is also one of the most reassuring facts for patients, clinicians, and policymakers: walking more is not associated with worsening back pain. Instead, the majority of the evidence suggests that walking is associated with a reduction in the reporting of back pain symptoms; improved function and disability; and a generally higher quality of life, even when coping with back pain. Further to these positive trends, there is accumulating evidence that as step counts go up, symptoms of back pain will reduce; there may also be a cut-off point beyond which back pain symptom prevalence benefits no longer increase, though this level of walking is quite high for chronic pain patients. Similarly, walking may also be linked to a higher perceived rate of global recovery from back pain. Importantly, for every step taken, walking is not just a passive neutral activity. A series of dose-dependent relationships have been observed between increasing levels of walking and increasing levels of physical, social, and psychological well-being, which have been shown to be independent of chronic back pain status. In general, walking, including higher amounts verging on formal exercise, is better for overall health and function, and it is good to walk more for those who can. For patients with back pain, the evidence appears to suggest that the more they can walk, the better they may feel in relation to some of the most difficult aspects of the problem. Such findings seem to suggest that all people walking try walking more, and that exercise and walking interventions targeting back pain should focus on adherence to the walking regimen and on elucidating the differential effects of walking at the patient's comfortable and maximal walking amounts. On balance, the implications of the findings are encouraging for efforts to get people walking, but care should be taken in stratifying recommendations for the use of walking as an exercise treatment, as some groups of patients may face specific issues or challenges related to the notion of walking more as an advised means of relief.

In this section, we discuss outcome measures that facilitate an understanding of the relationships between walking and back pain over time. These include global health and quality of life indices, as well as measures that facilitate tracking of participation in walking. In relation to back pain, medical quantitative and diagnostic indicators, as well as overall physical activity, binding effectors, and measures specific to the walking intervention being studied, are also pertinent.

5. Factors Affecting the Efficacy of Walking

In walking interventions carried out among patients, frequencies ranging from 3 to 7 times per week significantly reduced back pain. Both 3 to 5 times of walking per week may be effective in reducing pain. However, greater pain improvement is seen in people who walk 5 to 7 times weekly. According to a recent review, the duration of walking may range from a minimum of 20 min to a maximum of 90 min per occasion. Prolonged time spent walking (more than 30 min/day) may be a valid and effective pain reducer. Walking increases the aerobic capacity of patients with chronic low back pain, and according to the American College of Sports Medicine, 30 min of moderate-intensity exercise, most days beginning with 15 min if the patient is not used to physical exercise, can be efficient in reducing pain of patients with chronic low back pain. Therefore, this recently suggested recommendation may be in line with our recent review, where an improvement in low back pain among patients with chronic low back pain was observed for aerobic walking of at least 3 MET-hours/week (600 MET-minutes per week). As previously written, the rationale for less than 10 min rest intervals is in line with the available results, where less than 10 min walking produced variable effects, called small-to-moderate effect in low back pain in a cohort study of healthy people. In the clinical context, based on the three levels of evidence, further studies were needed to support the previous research suggesting that several walking velocities can be included in the training program and adopted as an alternative intervention in the management of low back pain based on the patients' preferences.

The efficacy of walking as an exercise to reduce back pain has been demonstrated in many cases. However, significant variability of the results exists according to the different study designs. The effectiveness of walking may be influenced by: amount of walking or frequency; duration; intensity; mode; posture in desk-based workers: sitting vs. standing vs. walking; characteristics of the sample (body mass index, age, time spent in sedentary behavior, and so on).

5.1. Frequency and Duration of Walking

This reduction in utilization of medical services is the gold standard/ultimate measure of public health benefit. The HEP+ repeated measures design and analysis expect at least one year of walking after the HEP if less than 50% permanently leave the healthcare system employment in the Intervention Plus Group. The use of medications may decrease over time as people walk longer. The longer the walking HEP continues and perhaps more.

The frequency and duration of walking associated with physical activity were explored in the articles included in this review, varying from walking sessions three to seven days a week to walking programs lasting six weeks to two years. Chronic health-related low back pain is a long-lasting condition. Decreased pain, increased strength, improved flexibility, and general health status are outcomes commonly assessed by healthcare professionals. Long-term walking may be preferred over shorter running or jogging sessions, especially for individuals with pain, as a physical activity recommendation as a treatment for appropriate people. Reducing the reliance on health care may be another long-term benefit of walking. Two of the three long-term walking studies reviewed showed improvements in pain over a 2-year duration, and in people with and without a history of pain over a 4.5-year duration. In the context of a 2.4-year group therapeutic walking intervention related to effectiveness, overutilization of health care decreased and satisfaction with treatment and walking were higher compared to unsupervised individual walkers at 2.3 years. To obtain economic and health care utilization benefits, walking regimens must be maintained for more than 2 years. It may take longer than a 2-year therapeutic walking center plus 2 years of home walks to further decrease or eliminate health care overuse.

5.2. Intensity of Walking

It seems that walking at an intensity of 3.5 mph (5.6 km/h) has medical benefits, while walking slowly is merely a physical activity. Increases in the level of activity and oxygen uptake can be achieved more quickly with an increased gait. The level of physical effort during long-distance running (a heart rate of 110 bpm) was attained by increasing the frequency and gait length to 2:9 in the research by Horst et al. The average speed (3 to 5 km/h) that may prevent or reduce lower-back pain has been associated by numerous possible anatomical and physiological changes in persons with lower-back pain. Reduced muscle tension, enhanced intervertebral disc nutrition, improved blood circulation and blood vessel density in the intervertebral disc, dermal and muscle, and reduced intradiscal pressures are mentioned in the studies. In summary, individuals with lower-back pain should walk at an intensity that does not make their pain worse. Based on AMBNRW guidelines, persons without lower-back pain should engage in moderate-intensity aerobic activity for a minimum of 30 min on five days a week.

The intensity of walking in relation to back pain has been examined in only a small number of empirical studies. It was observed that walking for a minimum of 30 min on one, two, or three occasions daily positively affected back pain. According to studies examining walking programs for persons with back pain, the optimal frequency of walking may not be particularly high, as walking even once a week was shown to result in less pain, better discs and nerve root circulation, and improved functioning. noted that walking affects the flexibility of the lumbar spine and strengthens the lumbar muscles, and as a result, relieves back pain. concluded that walking three to four times per week reduced the risk of lumbar radiculopathy. An eight-week program of walking four times at an average heart rate of 110 bpm resulted in a reduced pain score. Authors reported that individual walking plans in a study group with back pain decreased the pain intensity on a visual analogue scale from a value of 5 to 2 after 12 months. A Swiss study on the effects of walking on back pain is currently underway. Study participants are required to walk for 1 hour at a brisk pace every day. It is expected that walking will cause a significant improvement in back pain in study subjects; the study will be completed in November 2019. In addition to the frequency of walking, "off-loading packages" are included in the study plan as pain preventive measures.

5.3. Proper Walking Form

The phrases "good posture" and "proper form" are tossed around often in relation to walking. However, few—if any—sources supplying walking regimens provide descriptions of what these terms actually mean. Learning exercises is often done with both verbal and pictorial instructions to maximize effectiveness. Therefore, providing an overt objective provides a transparent standard from which to assess one's own walking form. By consensually defining these terms, what can emerge is a consistent method for using a low-impact form of exercise to alleviate lower back pain. In our opinion, walking to alleviate back pain should focus on maintaining a neutral spine in an attempt to focus purely on the muscle of interest, which is why the hands are placed on the front of the pelvis (anterior superior iliac spines) to provide objective feedback. In a standing position, the spine should have three natural curves. These curves are roughly shaped like the letter "S." Overall, walking endorses and improves the shock-absorbing capabilities of the spinal column, which may help attenuate back pain during activity. By not walking with proper form, the "shock" from striking the floor may travel up the kinetic chain to the inferior oblique abdominal muscles.

In the face of increased lower back pain, many people have begun to seek ways to alleviate their discomfort. In 2010, it was estimated that back pain represented nearly 12% of all physicians' visits, amounting to around 48 million visits annually. For people experiencing either chronic or subacute discomfort, walking is often advocated. This treatment is often regarded as beneficial, but most websites and sources provide only cursory information, such as suggested duration, surface, or incline. In this section, the most common misconception is likely to not walk with proper posture and form.

6. Combination Therapies for Back Pain

Combination of Physical Therapy and Medication Management The physical therapist can also work with the patient's physician to help the patient regulate the speed at which the medication is withdrawn by making adjustments in the walking program. Data shows that the best results in physical therapy happen with treatment sessions occurring twice a week. The main focus of the physical therapy sessions is to start a walking program and increase the patient's comfort while walking. As time goes on, the person is most commonly given specific exercises targeting the person's problem areas.

Combination Therapies Many researchers and clinicians report that combination therapies (more than one therapy used together) are best for patients with back pain. In studies of walking that have already been performed, most patients also received another form of therapy. The most common forms of therapy that patients combined with walking are other exercises, education, and medication management. The following section will discuss some basic guidelines for properly implementing walking in addition to medication management.

Back pain is a common medical complaint that affects many people and often results in referral to a physical therapist. Some evidence does support the idea that walking alone can be effective in reducing back pain. However, not all patients are ready for a walking program and it can sometimes be beneficial to start with other forms of exercise that may be easier for people who are just beginning to exercise or who have severe pain. In other patients, however, a walking program, sometimes in combination with physical therapy, is the best option.

6.1. Physical Therapy

In addition, the magnitude of change from baseline was similar between the LIFT and MED group at various time points. For example, in both groups, the proportion of participants with at least a 30-point change on the RMDQ was similar across the LIFT and MED group (49.5% LIFT group vs 48.5% MED, 12 months post-randomization). In a more recent trial, Saraux et al. compared a physical therapy plus walking intervention to a walking only intervention. It demonstrated large between group differences in pain and disability in favor of the combined intervention across follow-up. This evidence suggests that there may be a synergistic benefit to administering physical therapy concurrently with ambulatory exercise in back pain patients.

Clinical experts expressed a notion that when combined with physical therapy, walking would prove to be a highly effective treatment for back pain. Moreover, some of the trials discussed have implicated a synergistic effect between walking and physical therapy. For example, the treatment of the LIFT group was the same as the MED group excluding a physical therapy program. The primary outcome of interest was back pain and disability. This is the only rigorous trial to have observed the synergistic effects between physical therapy and walking. Although it is less methodologically sound when compared to a MED group, the LIFT group demonstrates a similar amount of overall recovery in both the 6 and 12-month follow-up.

6.2. Medication Management

Aside from NSAIDs, many other drugs, including antidepressants, cannabinoids, acetaminophen, and anti-seizure drugs, have been recommended for low back pain and neuropathic back pain. However, these treatments may not influence physiological variables improved in people with back pain, such as changes in muscle activation, mobility, gait speed, and pain latency, unless additional changes occur in other body systems. Given that walking can influence such variables, it may be that walking and medications have an additive or combined effect. However, further research is needed to determine this. Similarly, medications such as topical agents can be practical issues if they limit the ability to walk or the type of walking one engages in. Future research investigating the effects of walking in combination with medication management was recommended in the recent international promotion of walking guidelines.

4) Walking and back pain often accompany other comorbidities, such as physical or psychological impairments. Consequently, several treatment guidelines suggest combination (multimodal) treatments that may address more than one problem simultaneously. Medication management is included in such combination treatments. A detailed discussion on medication management is beyond the scope of this publication, especially since many medications were not included in the consensus statements from the studies of walking and back pain. However, three publications mentioned that walking

is an exercise modality that can be offered as a first-line non-pharmacological support for chronic pain. Additionally, both opioids and NSAIDs have side effects such as GI disturbances. The addition of exercise to anti-inflammatory drugs has also been suggested to be more effective for low back pain compared to anti-inflammatory drug use alone. This suggests that walking may be a beneficial part of a combination therapy for people with knee osteoarthritis.

7. Practical Recommendations for Incorporating Walking into Back Pain Management

Find the Positive: Incorporating Walking into a Back Pain Management Strategy Identify a walking goal and a reason for walking. For example, a goal may be "walk 1 mile" or "walk to the grocery store and back," and a reason may be for reducing stress or engaging with a friend. Start slowly and increase gradually. Establish a walking routine that is sustainable and progressive, choosing a duration and intensity that does not cause pain greater than a 3 on a 0-10 scale (0 = no pain, 10 = the worst pain imaginable). Provide your body with 24-48 hours of recovery before more walking, since pain after walking may not set in accurately until 24 hours post-walking.

Although walking symptoms could increase with pain, this doesn't necessarily mean individuals with low back pain are walking poorly or need to change their gait temporarily for pain relief. However, in conjunction with medical clearance, these individuals should seek clinical guidance from a healthcare provider who is proficient in gait analysis or works with running populations. For individuals with LBP interested in walking, clinicians may consider the following walking recommendations.

To increase the internal and external validity of these findings, high-quality research specifically designed to assess the effects of walking on individuals with low back pain should be conducted. This research should include improved walking-specific criteria, biofeedback, and the manipulation of walking prescriptions. Practitioners can provide general walking programs that gradually increase walking duration and intensity, especially for individuals with low back pain who may fear walking. Practitioners should also screen for walking biomechanics, balance, and cardiovascular and musculoskeletal fitness, and refer to a physiotherapist or exercise specialist if abnormalities are found.

Outcomes for incorporating walking into a back pain management strategy can be both positive (e.g., improved physical and psychological health) and negative (e.g., increased risk of injury). Creating a nuanced understanding of the therapeutic effects of walking among individuals with low back pain is critical for evidence-based practice.

Study Key Messages

7.1. Setting Realistic Goals

Musculoskeletal exercise interventions strive to enhance the ease through which activities can be performed while minimizing the activity itself. While high formal exercise compliance has important benefits in some areas, politicians have to vote for popular change, and not everyone wants to exercise. Advocating for walking or encouraging average daily step target increases creates an opportune moment to reset public and clinical expectations: the aim of physical activity is not to exceed the recommended weekly guidelines but to seek ways to minimize the barriers and maximize the ease with which the activities of daily life can be performed; namely, walking with reduced or no pain. If 10,000 steps is achievable without an increase in pain, great; if not, 5,000 will certainly suffice.

Seven days from now, is it feasible that those 10,000 steps will be achievable without pain? After all, you are a patient recovering from an injury or painful condition and should be taking it easy. Plans for increasing the average daily step count of people living with low back pain should be as specific and individualized as possible and set beyond the point of comfort, but short of injury, for that particular person on that particular day. The medications, imaging, biostimulations, and surgeries we recommend would not typically be achieved without some risk involved, but there is a definitive risk of failed intervention.

7.2. Gradual Progression of Walking Routine

In response to question 8, theme 2, it is notable to say that the paper has come to the conclusion, though using meta-analysis and several covariates. A comprehensive walking plan for low back pain demonstrates that walking at least twice a day on a daily basis may be helpful; however, the whole talking has to be a gradual one as it can increase the ability of a person.

In a recent qualitative review, levels of physical activity and exercise are recommended for people with a history of recurrent LBP. On this account, a gradual increase in walking may be helpful to stay active and meet daily activity levels. The participants stated that they found it easier to continue rather than to start a new walking routine, suggesting that gradual progression is preferred. Some studies have found that a slower increase in walking distance results in less pain and improved HRQoL, suggesting a possible therapeutic window. However, because participants seeking advice on a new walking routine may intuitively prefer gradual progression, this preference may have affected their perception of the intervention effect. It is still possible that this gradual approach may have benefits for reducing achievable objectives, minimizing the risk of overloading, and grounding early successes to maintain adherence and motivation. Given this evidence, a gradual approach was chosen when designing the walking program in the BoT-Back trial. Of important interest, future work could explore and understand the perspectives and opinions of individuals with LBP about the sources and walking parameters best suited for including in the walking program.

7.3. Consultation with Healthcare Providers

Walking may not be an ideal form of exercise for all people who are considering using it as a management strategy for their back pain. Just as there are certain people who might benefit from a walking program, there are also certain populations for whom beginning to walk regularly, particularly with back pain, might not be advisable. For example, if you have advanced cardiovascular disease, peripheral arterial disease, or severe vascular disease or are at significant risk of one of these conditions, increasing your activity level could increase your cardiovascular risk. In this instance, it may be best to walk only in a highly monitored clinical environment—in which case it would be considered chronic disease management.

Walking may not be right for some people.

Before beginning a walking program, particularly if you are attempting to treat your back pain through a daily walking habit, it's important to receive the go-signal from your healthcare provider. This is especially true if you have a history of chronic back pain, other chronic diseases or conditions, or if your back pain is the result of acute trauma. Your healthcare professional can help you determine the types of activities that would be safe and effective in your unique, individual case. They can also help you identify any red flags or important contraindications that indicate that walking may not be the best option for participating in physical therapy at that time. For example, if you're a person with an acute back injury, you may need to remain in bed for a certain period of time. Or you could have achieved a state of paralysis, which would also contraindicate walking as a therapy.

Consultation with your healthcare provider is advised.

8. Conclusion and Future Directions

During walking and complex interactions of anatomical structures, the mechanical forces responsible for the body and the prescription medication are also varied. A single medication approach is, therefore, doubtful to have the same effects. These early indications of studies are likely to be readily seen in studies concerning different states of the body. It is expected that the studies investigating the different types of walking and the effects of adaptation processes to the rehabilitation of the walking habits in chronic low back pain on the pain and effect will offer valuable input as well as the evaluation of walking as a long-term intervention method. The connection between walking and postural control and balance may also be the subject of the future studies. Although psychosocial determinants influencing efficiency and adjustment in pain are multifactorial, it was also recommended that patients suffering from depression or anxiety contribute to the walking features.

Walking is clearly indicated as an exercise that can be offered to patients struggling with back pain. Walking can contribute significantly to the relief of pain experienced by these individuals and also to providing them with a feeling of well-being. This is because walking facilitates the operation of any of the analgesic pathways that are considered the mechanisms of chronic pain. Because various sensorial inputs will be interacting with each other, the complexity of walking will require some processing of the central nervous system and motor output. Suggestions from these analytical protocols are required to be obtained. It is expected that studies analyzing the immediate and short-term effects will observe significant improvements, but studies involving longer evaluation periods might only be appropriate for more accurate evaluations.

8.1. Summary of Key Findings

Walking may be equivalent to psychosocial treatments regarding its ability to ameliorate pain, disability, psychological variables, and quality of life and superior to no exercise. Sex did not appear to influence the walking or control treatment outcomes for pain. In conclusion, walking did not worsen back pain and was as effective as psychosocial treatments for decreasing pain. A moderate to large reduction of pain was obtained after approximately 9 months of training in chronic LBP, and a moderate pain relief was observed over the short term (on average 2 months) in the acute stage. Evidence also suggested that frequent or regular walking (at least 3 times per week, on average) for reducing back pain had no disadvantages on disability. The majority of the samples were female, and the results of this review might be generalized only for a young to middle-age female population.

The treatment of chronic low-back pain (CLBP) is resistance training performed at 70 to 85 percent maximal strength. The evidence concerning the effects of walking on strength related to back pain is limited, but these results suggest that strength training may be superior to walking for decreasing back pain. In considering energy expenditure, walking performed at 3 mph or more appears to decrease lumbar pain by a moderate effect. However, in individuals who are sedentary, light to moderate levels of walking (either 1 to 2.9 mph or unknown speed) do not appear to ameliorate back pain. Clinically, the minimal level of walking speed to achieve a reduction in pain is unclear. Little evidence is available on the influence of walking on pain relief in pregnant women, older adults, and Latin people.

8.2. Areas for Further Research

• Walking type. No studies have attempted to realign biomechanics during walking, but seven clinical trials have observed the effects of altering step rate as a proxy strategy. This "gait retraining" has provided some early promise for pain reduction, with quite small improvements leading to clinically relevant changes for up to two weeks following the defined 20% increase. However, results in chronic back pain differ as not significant. Furthermore, a year-long walking intervention examining "low linear load" barefoot walking did not show greater effects on back pain compared to minimal footwear. This might propose that it is what goes on in the foot, rather than at the foot, that confers some of the benefits of walking. Another emphasis has been the effect of adding additional upper limb work into a walking program: adding Nordic walking poles to a ten-week walking program including between three and five physiotherapy sessions led to clinically relevant improvements in pain and functional disability up to 6 months post-intervention, including subgroup differences between normal and spondylolisthesis groups. Yet, back-related disability improved in the short-term (6 weeks), but not longer term, with the addition of weight vests into a three-times weekly resistance or interval-walking program conducted for ten weeks.

• Recruitment and adherence effect. Two studies evidenced suboptimal adherence after randomization to their walking interventions: a 12-week intervention showed a 60.6% rate, compared to a 70.2% adherence to a 6-week control, and another study found a trend for lower recruitment when the time commitment was higher.

The Benefits of Walking for Relieving Back Pain

1. Introduction to Back Pain and Walking

Our back supports the entire weight of the body that gets put on it, and that is why it is one of the most strained parts of our body. This may be as a result of carrying heavy weight, sitting in a bad posture the entire day due to a desk job or sleeping on a tough mattress. This can result in an individual having severe pain in the back. Sometimes, however, back pain when walking can be as a result of an underlying health concern. Walking can relieve back pain by reducing stress on the joints in the spine, including reducing pressure on the disc between your vertebrae and distributing more nutrients into the cartilage of the joints. So when patients are advised to start moving more, walking is one of the first activities to be recommended as it is easy on the back and has plenty of pain-relieving benefits.

People often think the best way to deal with back pain is staying in bed. While bed rest can help provide some relief, there are specific activities that can further help reduce back pain, and one prominent one is walking. Researchers have found that walking is as effective as any other activities like exercising and physical therapy in reducing pain and improving the quality of life of people with chronic lower back pain. If you are too skeptical to give this a try, I'll suggest you read on, to understand how walking affects back pain and how quickly you can get the benefits from walking for back pain. Here, we are going to discuss the relationship between back pain and walking, why walking can help with your back pain, and how to start walking for this purpose.

1.1. Understanding Back Pain

Research is continuing to be developed about back pain, but it is perhaps more interesting to consider the impact of back pain. Back pain not only affects an individual by population size, but it also affects in perhaps the most profound ways. It affects quality of life by disrupting sleep, taking away the ability to work, and is prevalent in soldiers who have been abroad. Even with over $240 billion of annual cost spent on treating back pain, this issue is not a regional issue, but a global one. When back pain touches nearly everyone, it is important to look at it in a new light as perhaps people have been looking to approaches that have not improved the solution of this growing issue.

Back pain is a condition that can range from mildly annoying to an unbearable debilitating condition. It can be sourced from muscle strains, disc herniations, facet joint disease, arthritis, osteoporosis, or even lifestyle choices. It can include symptoms such as stiffness, aching, burning, sharp, traveling pain into the extremities, and even weakness. In the United States alone, over forty-five million people are affected by it. And of that forty-five million, there are half of those who live with a type of back pain that is not resolved within one year. And even more astounding is that back pain is one of the most common reasons most individuals visit the doctor and results in losing income.

1.2. Benefits of Walking for Back Pain Relief

Beyond the direct back pain relieving benefits of walking, the act of walking can be considered a biomechanical treatment for existing back pain, as well as an insurance policy to prevent future pain. Walking also encourages weight loss to relieve the pressure on the joints, and gives the back improved postural alignment, balance and coordination with movement. A walking schedule can be of critical importance for anyone with occasional or chronic back pain to prevent an 'abdominal attack' of lower back pain. The main core muscles targeted when walking are the same ones that help strengthen the lower back, and the naturally aligned posture encouraged by walking provides further back relief, decreasing the pressure on the discs and the risk of causing damage and further back injury.

When people experience back pain, the large stabilizing muscles in the back weaken and our muscles tense up as we try to guard against further pain. Exercise can help to strengthen weakened muscles, while walking helps to reintegrate the muscles that have tensed up. In restoring the natural walking motion people once had or were meant to have, many find that they can walk their way out of a great deal of back pain, if not all. On a physiological level, walking is excellent cardiovascular exercise that helps to pump fresh oxygenated blood around the body while expelling toxins and waste. This blood flow is especially important in the lumbar region, which relies on continual flow of blood and nutrients for its health and recovery. Psychological benefits are also realized from walking, as it releases feel good endorphins and gives people a sense of freedom and confidence that they can actively manage their chronic back pain.

There are many reasons why walking can help people who suffer with back pain. The physical and postural benefits of walking alleviate existing back pain and provide protection for the future, while other benefits provide further support for people with chronic back pain.

2. Anatomy of the Spine and Muscles Involved

Spinal anatomy, when looking at the full-spine from the side or front, is shown to be composed of vertebrae, bony segments separated by a soft intervertebral disk. Surrounding the vertebral bodies and intervertebral disks are multiple muscles concentrated in the back. Muscles serve many roles in spinal mechanics, including the movement and control of the spine in multiple directions.

The back is a general term describing the portion of the body between the base of the neck and the top of the buttocks. It includes a number of interconnected parts, including the spine, the musculature surrounding the spine, and the joints that connect each vertebra. Adequate understanding of these connections is critical to understanding not just why walking aids in the relief of back pain, but to understand the physical forces which act on the structures and how to use those forces to one's advantage. This paper addresses this holistic view of the fundamental connections between the primary structures associated with back pain, the actions which reproduce pain in patients, and why walking is useful in the treatment of back pain. It does not attempt to address a wide range of remedial physical therapy options for back pain and, most notably, it does not address a wide variety of medications and treatments often suggested by a medical doctor for treating back and leg pain suggested by the medical doctor who refer the back pain and walking patients.

2.1. Structure of the Spine

Thus, loss of disc height is a good measure of the shortening effect of load bearing. This loss has the power to increase in a 24-hour period and promote early low back pain. Pain can be viewed as protective; nociceptors are the pain reception neurons found in the annulus fibrosus and posterior longitudinal ligament of lumbar discs. They send their nerve endings to healthy (non-degenerated) nucleus pulposus and a large portion of the outer annulus fibrosus. Increased pressure on disc structures impinges on these nociceptors, which then activate large spinal nerve fibers that transmit the pain message to the brain. Postural abnormalities or forward head posture increases the pressure and can cause disc impingement, which results in pain transmission. Organic changes can develop over time and can morph into radiating or referred pain and even nutrient deficiencies to the nerve roots as vascular-nerves are compressed. This, if it happens, can result in peripheralization of pain. Regarding literature that pain subsides when walking, it can be concluded that walking activates muscle activity, influencing regional blood circulation and lymph flow in the lower extremity and paraspinal muscles. However, it should be stated that this study does have limitations, such as there are only twenty articles analyzed. For the purpose of this review, the number of articles found is too low.

The spine is the structure in the body that allows a person to stand, bend, and twist, as well as protect the spinal cord. Each vertebra or bone of the spine is a separate structure and has two sets of facet joints. These joints are what allow the spine to perform these movements and are lubricated in the same way as the knee and hip joints. Consequently, hyaline cartilage lines the bone ends and produces synovial fluid. The spine is also supported by structures such as the intervertebral disc that has different roles when compared with the joint. Therefore, the disc allows for side bending and rotation to take place. The special shape of the vertebrae, when combined with the disc and tension of the various ligaments, helps to form a canal that protects the spinal cord of a person. This canal is called the spinal canal. The transfer of loads from the upper body to the lower body is also the role of the spine. This is completed by the vertebral bodies and the intervertebral discs.

2.2. Key Muscles Involved in Walking and Back Support

Three different types of muscles are involved in the process of walking. While contributory muscles shorten and lengthen between the pelvis and the femur to provide balance, power, and smooth momentum and are the most involved in determining gait and running symmetry and grace, the supportive muscles that position the pelvis such as the quadratus lumborum, the piriformis, and the hip adductors, and those involved in creating force and tension such as the iliopsoas, adductor longus, and tensor fasciae latae, play a considerable role in providing balance and relief to the back.

Many muscles are engaged in the act of walking, and by virtue of their extensive anatomical locations, the muscles around the hips and pelvis play a surprisingly considerable role in supporting the spine and the muscles that control lower-back motion. Indeed, the muscles of the legs, hips, and pelvis are interconnected with the deep muscles of the back that feel sore when we have a bad back. This relationship may explain why such a high percentage of individuals who walk a lot and walk fast do not have lower-back pain. As the legs and hips move in a natural, strong, graceful fashion, the muscles of the lower back can gently twist, bend, and flex, which improves blood flow and provides nutrients and oxygen and removes waste products from the deep tissues in the lower back. This is one reason why walking is a top recommendation for physical therapy and rehabilitation for sore backs. It is also why slowing down the natural gait with the wrong type of footwear, entering a poorly designed gym class, or striking the treadmill too hard can cause as many back problems as it resolves.

3. Proper Walking Techniques

Techniques are key. When we are forced to walk on our two hind feet, the stresses to the many components of the lower extremity increases dramatically. Hence, research indicates that the average person would feel tired after only 8 to 10 miles of walking on bare feet, but could easily exceed 30 miles and still feel up to walking there later when wearing properly designed walking shoes. The concept is simple. The exact same principle applies to the "art of walking." While an average person might be able to walk for a certain distance, a person with a properly aligned and functioning lower extremity might be able to walk much further and with a higher level of efficiency partially due to the decreased potential for injury.

Proper Pathology. As always, we must consider and compensate for different problems and conditions that may already exist. If you suffer from general muscular tension or tightness – or specific myofascial syndromes – you may need more than just a simple stark-up support placed a size 9 shoe off the ground. Simple physical appeal. Proper walking also has an appealing aesthetic effect on posture, since the foot inverts when it hits the ground, the foot's support, the hip is encouraged to abduct, producing that "looking good" walk.

Just as high-tech exercise equipment, training programs, and workout gear have become more available, it has become easier and more tempting to forget about the simplest tool for gaining and preserving physical health:

walking. Of course, not all walking techniques render the same benefits. The way you walk and the surface you walk on affects how much impact and stress is placed upon the muscles, ligaments, and skeletal system, and can either increase or decrease your risk of low back pain and related problems.

Effectively walk your way out of back pain!

3.1. Posture and Alignment

Walking with good posture and alignment can provide significant back pain relief. The secrets of optimal posture are that each body part is recruited into the tasks for which it is best designed. For walking, this means being in a position in which the strong muscles of the core are well-coordinated and working together to stabilize the spine and pelvis (femur, ribcage, and shoulder). Try to align the tip of the shoulder with the outer 3rd of the hip, the knee with the toes, and aim to walk with the feet parallel (toes are facing slightly inward at 10 o'clock-2 o'clock). Use this "strong stance" or "balance-stance" as your walking position and aim to train muscles to support this. Attempt to make the pelvis a "three wheel drive" by using the 4 muscles that connect the pelvis to the spine to stabilize the base of the spine into a "neutral" position (standing straight in good posture). These muscles are the transverse abdominis, rectus abdominis, and obliques (the inside and outside of the two diagonal muscles). Unless necessary for an additional therapeutic challenge, avoid holding a leveler on the back as most find that it no longer allows them to contract the deep postural muscles for stabilizing the base of the spine and it can shift the contractile demand away from the stronger muscles of the core to the shoulders, which are not adapted for that load. Keep smaller weights ordered by carrying in your hands or invest in a weighted vest. Start with no more than 2.5-5lbs and add 1lb a week as strength improves to reduce 20-75% (from normal body weight) of cumulative impact over the course of the walks.

Walking is good for your cardiovascular system and can be a good lockdown activity, as it is essential exercise and can be done around your home. It is suitable for adults of all ages. It increases your heart rate, strengthens your muscles, is good for bone health, and can be uplifting. Walking outdoors has the added provision of fresh air and exposure to natural light for bone health. To increase your walking experience or to help overcome a plateau, the following guide describes how to manually control pace, base of support, training distance, and intensity beyond maintaining good posture and alignment. It has to be easy and non-stressful to integrate these recommendations.

3.2. Footwear and Walking Surfaces

Walking surfaces. The artificial surfaces of gyms welcome walkers to climate-controlled, smooth and accident-free environments, but concrete, macadam, and turf walking surfaces present opportunities to access the potential mental health benefits of green exercise. Green exercise describes the diverse ways in which exercising in natural environments can contribute to healthy living. Research reveals that walking on different surfaces can affect the muscles used by the body in various ways. The body responds to walking on soft ground (like a turf walking trail) with a slower walking speed and generally smaller steps. This means that you will take more steps than if you were walking on a hard surface. The Achilles tendon and calf muscles will also have to stretch and contract to an even greater degree. Although we know very little about how the surface we walk on may affect the development of LBP, it is likely that softer surfaces could contribute to the health of the intervertebral discs in much the same way that they do the knees.

Proper footwear. Your feet support the entire weight of your body as you walk, which means that the comfort and cushioning your shoes afford play a major role in not just your capacity to exercise or commute by walking, but also your back health. Given the array of different foot types and body biomechanics, the ideal shoe for you may differ from someone else. Generically speaking, it is important to ensure that you have adequate arch support and shock absorption in your shoes. You are more likely to experience the benefits of supportive footwear if you switch to flat shoes without heels. Heels on shoes cause changes in the curvature of your spine and can even apply increased pressure to your lower discs.

Section 3.2. Footwear and Walking Surfaces

4. Designing a Walking Program for Back Pain Relief

Customize your plan of treatment: Numerous studies have successfully administered exercise programs to groups of people, and the programs have improved over time, resulting in better outcomes. Your program should reflect your personal circumstances, such as the severity of your back pain, your existing level of physical activity, the amount of time you have available to walk, and your personal walking abilities. For example, if you are sedentary, you may need to begin more gradually than an individual who performs regular high-impact aerobic exercise.

Monitor improvements over time: Track your progress, such as walking time, using various benchmarks across the day or week. Before deciding if the walking is successful, participants in the training studies measured themselves to determine if feedback was working. In a clinical setting, a physical therapist or other health professional may help you establish goals and monitor your success.

Focus on acute changes in the back: Keep tabs on how your back feels as you begin walking. While it's usual to have an increase in symptoms when you first start walking, you should try to limit intensity within this threshold so that the increase in pain quickly decreases.

Lay out a plan for achieving your exercise goals: For example, your first goal could be to walk for 15 minutes without increasing your low back pain. Once this is achieved, the next goal is to add another two or three minutes of walking to your routine. After that, the pace will slow as you gradually work to increase your daily walking time. This approach has been used in exercise trials with people who have chronic low back pain and have been found to be useful in achieving long-term exercise goals.

Create a walking program: It's possible to start walking to help relieve back pain by simply walking more and standing less throughout the day. However, it may be more beneficial to start from scratch and design a walking program that is specifically designed to reduce low back pain. This technique has been evaluated in multiple studies, including trials with as few as four or eight weekly sessions. A well-structured program can help reduce a person's impairment when they hurt their back and begin to continue walking.

4.1. Setting Realistic Goals

Because most walking programs are flexibility, aerobic fitness, and strength exercise programs, it's important to understand how to structure warm-up and cool-down strategies. A warm-up is important to increase blood flow to the muscles, increase the core body temperature, and increase the heart rate. Warm-up activities can include stretching, walking slowly, and doing range-of-motion activities. The cool-down is important to help prevent stiffness and soreness after exercising. A cool down can be a short period during which you walk slowly and perform a few exercises to help you stretch. The amount of time varies based on your pre-exercise heart rate. The most important point is to do both exercises and walking at a low rate of speed. As there is no equipment necessary for most of these exercises, they can be performed on the same day as many of your other walking program exercises that use exercise balls.

Establishing realistic goals is an important part of your walking program. Your healthcare professional will help you set specific goals, the first of which may be to walk to the end of your block. In time, walking a mile may become possible, and then perhaps longer distances. If you set achievable objectives, you'll be likely to stick with your program. Being realistic in setting goals doesn't mean setting the bar too low; it's important to set a goal that is challenging, but that also takes into account your current level of fitness and your health status. Reaching the milestones of your walking program will help keep you motivated as your progress verifies your hard work.

4.2. Progressive Overload and Rest

Rest is a vital component when using this return in the program. As stated earlier, a lack in response to the recommended walking programs may be possibly, in part, put down to a failure to progressively overload in a wave-like pattern. This management plan could be attempted with information on managing unmade psychological predisposition to chronicity and sensitivities clearly presented to the individual in the form of a client educational handout.

If a structured program mainly implements walking to help relieve back pain, then progressive overload – a systematic increase in walking demands – will have to be utilized to help manage ongoing symptoms, while still allowing regular planned improvements in fitness. So long as the concept of 'progressive overload' is adhered to, the principle of 'more is better' is maintained, and blame is not laid entirely on the development of symptoms on average walking speed or type of surface, this increase should not unduly provoke symptoms. Walking time can be cautiously increased, starting anywhere near the bottom of the range and gradually working up to the top end of the time the individual has available and contains rest time within it. At the end of the increasing symptom-free time individuals would then walk at the higher time for two weeks (14 days) of this being week two and not the starting two weeks of the new time. Following on from this an increase to walking up to the pain with at least 2 rest periods is introduced.

5. Incorporating Stretching and Strengthening Exercises

It's important to stress that you shouldn't experience any pain when doing these exercises. They should just feel like various degrees of a stretch, never reaching the point of discomfort. If any of these exercises cause or increase pain, try doing them for a shorter amount of time or reducing the effort you put into the movement. If you haven't already, talk to your doctor or a physical therapist about what type of exercise is the best for you specifically before starting a new workout routine. Speaking from experience, I can tell you that just walking alone often isn't going to completely resolve low back pain. But I can empathize when you don't feel good. The only thing you want to do is feel better. Adding these exercises to your daily walks might be the best place to start.

To boost the relief that walking can provide, you might want to include some simple stretching and strengthening exercises. A big review published in the peer-reviewed journal JAMA Internal Medicine found that combining walking with exercises that improve strength and flexibility was more effective than just walking or just doing strengthening or flexibility exercises. The authors of the review stressed the need for coordinated, holistic health advice and management for low back pain that focuses on the physical, psychological, and environmental factors that influence chronic pain and disability. DeLorme stretching is a way of applying deep pressure during stretching, which can yield better results than regular stretching exercises, McKenzie says.

5.1. Stretching for Back Pain Relief

Here are the 10 best stretching exercises: chest stretch, neck side stretch, neck stretch, upper back stretch with hands shoulder-width apart, upper back stretch with a resistance band, outer thigh and glute stretch, hamstring stretch, hip flexor stretch, and calf stretch. As per noted by Harvard Medical School, it is crucial to consult with a doctor and to make sure you do not have any health problems that would prevent you from exercising. It is worth pointing out that the stretching exercises can be easily adapted to one's physical condition. You should adjust stretching exercises to your own abilities and perform 2 to 3 times to overall tolerance; make 5 to 15 repetitions in each; don't make sudden movements and instead stretch gently.

Back pain is a common problem that can often be relieved by walking. It is worth asking, however, if other actions can further improve one's walk and thus help prevent future discomfort. Put simply, stretching exercises can contribute to relieving back pain even more. Back stretching exercises enable you to stretch in multiple directions, including the forward, backward, and sideways directions, increasing your flexibility. Moreover, tension in the muscles can be reduced with stretching exercises, which results in reduced discomfort. All in all, stretching exercises contribute to improving your walk more than physical activity alone. Stretching exercises can be done at home all by yourself, before or after your walk, or while doing other light physical activity.

5.2. Strengthening Exercises for the Core and Back Muscles

Strengthening exercises targeted towards strengthening the core muscles can have a big impact on the level of back pain one has, as the muscles can also protect the back from certain aggravating movements. Some of the muscles clumped under the "italic" lumbar spine and hip muscles "italic" are: the erector spinae, multifidus, obliques, transversalis, rectus abdominis, quadratus lumborum, hamstrings, iliacus, iliocostalis, and the intertransversarii. Exercises that can help fortify these muscles include: hamstring stretch, cat stretch, pelvic tilt, leg raises, plank, the upper back flexion, curl-ups, and leg lifts. A physiotherapist or exercise physiologist can help tailor an exercise program targeting these muscle groups so as to not overexert oneself. A comprehensive approach needs to consider the symptoms and also the cause of pain.

In the presence of back pain, these muscles often become weak. With quick and effective treatments, research has shown that these muscles get deactivated and become fatty. With the loss of muscle strength, the spine becomes less stable. Hence, one will experience pain earlier (i.e., less work time before one experiences pain), less stamina, and will fatigue more quickly. Sitting in a wrong way and performing heavier work can further destabilize the spine and decrease muscle strength, increasing the onset of back pain.

The core muscles start from the mid-thighs up to the shoulders. These muscles travel across the front, sides, and back. They play a big role in maintaining an upright posture and moving the spine in multiple directions. The muscles of the low back also play the same role.

Core and back strengthening exercises

6. Other Tips and Considerations

Listen to the Body Individuals should strive to listen to their body and exercise at a level defined by their body's condition and tolerance. Aches are common, as is some degree of muscle fatigue, after an exercise session. Individuals should strive to distinguish between "good" pain (also called "delayed-onset muscle soreness" following exercise) and "bad" pain ("bad" pain increases during exercise, while "good" pain decreases; if there is any question, individuals should consult with their personal medical providers). Similarly, when walking, some individuals might experience some soreness or fatigue from using muscles and the "new" activity. Starting slowly and listening to the body can help avoid injuries or soreness as the body adapts to exercise.

1. Hydration. Drinking water helps keep the body well-hydrated to support the health of all tissues and decrease the risk of muscle cramping. 2. Nutrition. Eating a nutritious diet is beneficial for maintaining a healthy weight and providing the nutrients needed for optimal bodily function. Limiting processed, high-sugar, and high-fat foods may help prevent inflammation and support overall health and wellness. 3. Sunscreen. Walking outside has a higher risk of overexposure to the sun. Applying an appropriate SPF sunscreen may prevent sunburn and skin damage. 4. Gait and Posture. As walking for back pain is intended to help improve gait and posture, it may be helpful to pay attention to the movement of the body while

walking. Practicing body awareness can help recipients know when they are not maintaining proper alignment, which can be corrected in the moment. 5. Walk with Supervision. For individuals with severe back pain or current inability to safely walk on their own, walking with a partner or practitioner may be beneficial. Walking with a partner can also add social support and increase motivation to continue.

- About 15.5 cups (or 124 ounces) of fluid daily for men - About 11.5 cups (or 92 ounces) of fluid daily for women. Stretch across a 16-hour day, as humans should consume fluids over the course of the entire day. The type of fluids one consumes in a day heavily relies on their overall nutrition. Here's a simple technique to obtain hydration data via behavior monitoring: jot down what you eat and drink, and then sum the amount of fluids consumed over a 16-hour day. Any person, on any mission to include more walking to mitigate back pain, should consider what they consume to maintain healthful benefits. Hydration guidelines outlined to maintain a basic level of health enhance the likelihood of further benefits from walking. Every person plays an active role in their life by taking in the necessary nutrients to help their tissue and muscles recover more efficiently and move towards improvements in health through walking.

The body is an interconnected machine, and the systems within it are influenced by one another. For example, in order for muscles and tissues to function at their best, they require proper nutrients. The intervertebral discs in the spine, and the muscle tissue throughout the posterior aspect of the body, are influenced by the systemic environment created by the body. If fluids are not maintained, the body cannot function at its best, and one of the most basic systems affected is hydration. The overall reliability and health of the tissues designed to support appropriate movement of the body are fundamentally influenced by intake of necessary nutrients. Proficiency in consuming enough water is essential to moving towards improved quality of life and walking more to mitigate back pain. A registered dietitian or nutritionist may be an asset for some populations. Currently, ADA states the amount of water one needs to consume depends both on sex and how much they sweat, but the organization's general recommendation is:

6.2. Listening to Your Body

Breaking up your walking sessions can make it feel more achievable. If you experience any pain in your back and walking causes you to have more pain, chances are you may be walking for too long, or your steps may be too long. In cases like these, you will likely need to cut back on walking, stop walking, or rest before walking again. If you walk up to a point where it becomes painful, take a break. If a longer break is needed, don't hesitate, rest, or stop walking for the day. Dig into the depths of your body signals and see what your body really needs.

While your body can provide great relief of what works and doesn't work, it's important to listen to your body when it is giving you feedback. Remember that you are the only one that truly knows what you are and are not feeling. Additionally, there are subtle signals and cues to both listen for and to adjust accordingly, that include being tired, to having sore muscles. If your muscles are sore, do not push yourself to do more, instead, listen to your body and stop or at least slow down. Walking at a pace that doesn't tire you out, doing a reasonable time, and engaging regularly on a daily basis can help improve your strength, flexibility, and overall endurance.

7. Conclusion and Summary

Although the results of this essay in terms of back pain are somewhat specific, the benefits are less clear. It continues a systematic review exploring the effect of "all-rounded" walking on back symptoms in the chronic lifespan. Even though national directives endorse training as the "best choice" for LBP consideration and walking is indeed the most studied of these trainings, "walking on its own" could provide perceptions that would not be standardized involving other methods. Further explorations may assist people in isolating the scales of those that live at home and are more sociable. Want to become the general public.

In conclusion, chronic back pain in the form of LBP imposes restrictions on specific physical activities and restrictions due to many athletes needing surgical interventions. Although exercise has been placed as the top recommendation by national guidelines, including walking being one of the most common forms of exercise, a handful of studies have examined walking in isolation. The most significant result of this review was that walking increases flexion excitement. It helps relieve back pain, enhance the production of endorphins, improve the stress of neurotransmitters, enhance pain pulses launched from the brain, improve levels of stiffness in the person's back, improve flexibility level of the person, and help with people sleeping when cadenced late.

7.1. Recap of Key Points

- If done at a comfortable pace and on level ground, walking is a safe and effective way to relieve the symptoms of lower back pain and prevent its onset, based on scientific evidence. - There are several reasons why walking is so beneficial for keeping back pain at bay. Walking can strengthen the muscles that support the back, increase blood flow and nutrients to the spine to facilitate the healing process, reduce pain and inflammation, lubricate joints and reduce stiffness, increase flexibility and range of motion, improve posture, and above all, clear your head by inducing the release of pain-relieving chemicals called endorphins in the brain. - Incorporate walking into your daily routine either in one go or by splitting it into shorter walks in the morning, afternoon, and evening for a minimum of 150 minutes a week. Walk at a brisk pace where your breathing rate becomes harder, but you can still talk. Exercises to improve strength and flexibility should also be added. It has not been scientifically confirmed whether walking alone is more effective than walking combined with strength and flexibility training. Walking is most effective when repeated regularly and lifelong. Keep in mind to practice good walking posture and wear supportive and comfortable shoes.

Key Takeaways:

7.2. Future Directions for Research

Gait kinematics and the condition of neuromuscular systems are used to evaluate stress and thereby discomfort in individuals who walk every day. Research in this implies that we learn about the activity of the muscles of the trunk and hip in finding out which muscles behave in what situations during walking. Research in this area will aid us in choosing participation indices. Research on EMG is also necessary. In order to determine the most effective way to perform lumbar stabilization exercises, we need to investigate the muscles of the proximate limbs. Muscles can be prioritized according to their importance in gait. The evolved muscles that are instrumental in stabilizing the lumbar spine synergistically during the stance phase can be assessed to ensure greater efficiency in performing pelvic and core stability work. In an effort to evaluate the chance of a subsequent occurrence of pain, it should be examined whether an alteration can increase the degree of stress and discomfort for the occurrences of low back pain in populations with a history of LBP. This is also an open avenue of research in a setting or client dealing with ergonomics. This makes it easier to measure discomfort levels in future studies.

It is important to continue developing and diversifying knowledge about walking as a curative activity that relieves back problems. The range of questions to be worked on is introduced in this chapter. Research in biomechanics is needed. The questions emphasize the need for a habitual gait biomechanical research using 3-D. In order to help people with back pain learn about how to handle it during their daily lives, we must find the rapid modifications in the gait that can occur when someone delivers an occasional or daily dose of the walking programs reported in the literature.